UNLOCKING THE PRITIKIN DIET

Science-Based Strategies for Improved Well-Being and Weight

Dr. Raymond F. Bernard

TABLE OF CONTENTS

CHAPTER 1

Introduction to the Pritikin Diet

In the world of diets and nutrition, the Pritikin Diet stands out as a pioneer in promoting health and well-being through dietary choices. Its origins can be traced back to the vision and dedication of Nathan Pritikin, a man who sought to revolutionize how we think about food and its impact on our bodies. This chapter is your gateway to understanding the essence of the Pritikin Diet, its core principles, and the profound health benefits it offers.

The Genesis of Pritikin Diet: A Visionary's Pursuit of Health

Nathan Pritikin, the visionary behind the Pritikin Diet, was not a doctor or nutritionist by profession, but rather an inventor and engineer. His journey into the world of health and nutrition was personal. In the 1950s, at the age of 42, Pritikin faced a daunting health crisis. He was diagnosed with heart disease, a condition that typically carried a grim prognosis at the time.

Rather than passively accepting his fate, Pritikin embarked on a remarkable quest to understand and transform his health. His first step was to immerse himself in scientific literature on nutrition, physiology, and heart disease. What he discovered was revolutionary. He learned that diet played a pivotal role in heart health, and he was determined to put this knowledge into practice.

The Core Principles of the Pritikin Diet

The Pritikin Diet is founded on a few fundamental principles, each of which plays a crucial role in promoting health and longevity:

1. **Low Fat, High Fiber**: One of the cornerstone principles of the Pritikin Diet is the restriction of dietary fat. Pritikin believed that excessive fat consumption, particularly saturated and trans fats, was a major contributor to heart disease and other chronic illnesses. Instead, he advocated for a diet rich in high-fiber foods like fruits, vegetables, whole grains, and legumes.

2. **Plant-Based Emphasis**: The Pritikin Diet leans heavily toward plant-based eating. This means that the majority of your food should come from plant sources, such as fruits, vegetables, nuts, seeds, and grains. Animal products like meat and dairy are limited, especially those high in saturated fat.

3. **Moderate Protein**: While the diet is primarily plant-based, it doesn't exclude protein. However, the protein sources recommended are lean, such

as poultry, fish, and plant-based alternatives like tofu and beans. This moderation ensures you get the protein your body needs without excessive saturated fat.

4. **Portion Control**: Understanding portion sizes is vital to the Pritikin Diet. It's not just about what you eat but also how much. Portion control helps manage calorie intake and prevents overeating.

5. **Whole, Unprocessed Foods**: Pritikin emphasized the importance of consuming whole and

minimally processed foods. Highly processed foods, with their added sugars, unhealthy fats, and artificial ingredients, were discouraged. Instead, the focus was on foods as close to their natural state as possible.

The Health Benefits of the Pritikin Diet

Perhaps the most compelling reason to consider the Pritikin Diet is its track record of delivering significant health benefits. It's not merely a diet for weight loss, although it can be remarkably effective for shedding excess pounds. The Pritikin Diet also has a profound impact on heart health, diabetes management, and overall well-being.

1. **Heart Health**: Pritikin's personal journey with heart disease spurred his passion for heart health. By adhering to the principles of the Pritikin Diet, individuals have experienced dramatic reductions in cholesterol levels, blood pressure, and inflammation – all key factors in heart disease. For

many, this diet has been a lifeline, helping them avoid heart surgery and medications.

2. **Weight Loss**: The Pritikin Diet is known for its ability to promote sustainable weight loss. By emphasizing low-calorie-density foods and portion control, individuals can achieve and maintain a healthy weight. Unlike crash diets, this approach isn't about quick fixes but rather long-term well-being.

3. **Diabetes Management**: For those with diabetes, the

Pritikin Diet can be a game-changer. Its focus on high-fiber, low-fat foods helps stabilize blood sugar levels. Many individuals with type 2 diabetes have reduced or even eliminated their need for medication through this diet.

4. **Overall Well-Being**: Beyond specific health conditions, the Pritikin Diet contributes to a sense of vitality and well-being. People report increased energy, better sleep, and a heightened sense of mental clarity. This isn't just about

adding years to your life but about adding life to your years.

The Enduring Legacy of Nathan Pritikin

To truly appreciate the Pritikin Diet, it's essential to recognize the man behind the movement. Nathan Pritikin's journey from heart disease patient to health pioneer is a testament to the transformative power of lifestyle choices. His dedication to scientific inquiry, coupled with his practical approach to nutrition, laid the foundation for a movement that has touched countless lives.

Pritikin's legacy extends far beyond the diet itself. He opened the Pritikin Longevity Center in the 1970s, providing a place for individuals to immerse themselves in the principles of the diet and experience its benefits firsthand. His work has inspired a community of health professionals, chefs, and advocates who continue to promote the Pritikin lifestyle.

Conclusion

In this introductory chapter, you've been introduced to the Pritikin Diet, a dietary approach rooted in science and driven by a passion for health. As you delve deeper into the subsequent chapters, you'll gain a comprehensive understanding of how to implement the Pritikin Diet in your own life, discover delicious and nutritious recipes, and learn from the inspiring success stories of individuals who have transformed their health through this remarkable approach. The journey you're embarking on isn't just about food; it's about embracing a new way of living that has the power to enhance your well-being for years to come.

CHAPTER 2

Understanding the Science Behind the Pritikin Diet

Welcome to Chapter 2, where we dive deep into the scientific underpinnings of the Pritikin Diet. If you've ever wondered why this diet is so effective in promoting health and well-being, you're about to find out. We'll explore the fascinating connections between nutrition, physiology, and the principles that form the bedrock of the Pritikin Diet.

The Pritikin Approach to Science

Nathan Pritikin was not a scientist or medical doctor by training, but he had an engineer's mind for problem-solving. When he was diagnosed with heart disease in the 1950s, he embarked on a personal quest to understand the mechanics of his ailment and how lifestyle, particularly diet, could influence it.

What Pritikin found in his extensive research was nothing short of groundbreaking. He discovered that heart disease, often considered an inevitable consequence of aging, was primarily driven by lifestyle factors, with diet playing a central role. This was a paradigm shift in the world of medicine and nutrition, and it laid the foundation for the Pritikin Diet.

The Role of Nutrition in Health

Central to the Pritikin Diet is the idea that what we eat profoundly affects our health. At its core, the diet recognizes that food is more than just fuel; it's information for our bodies. Every morsel we consume communicates with our cells, impacting everything from our energy levels to our risk of chronic diseases.

Understanding Calories and Nutrients

Before we delve into the specifics of the Pritikin Diet, let's clarify some fundamental concepts.

1. **Calories**: Calories are units of energy found in food. We need them for our body to function, but excess calories can lead to weight gain. The Pritikin Diet emphasizes calorie density, focusing on foods with fewer calories per gram, which helps control

calorie intake without leaving you hungry.

2. **Macronutrients**: These are the three major nutrients our bodies require in large amounts:

   - **Carbohydrates**: Carbs are the body's primary energy source. Pritikin advocates for complex carbohydrates found in whole grains, fruits, and vegetables.

   - **Proteins**: Proteins are essential for growth, repair, and overall body function. The Pritikin Diet encourages lean protein sources, both animal-based (like poultry and fish) and plant-based (like beans and tofu).

- **Fats**: While fat is necessary, the Pritikin Diet promotes low-fat choices. Saturated and trans fats, often found in processed and animal-based foods, are minimized, and healthy fats from sources like nuts, seeds, and avocados are emphasized.

3. **Micronutrients**: These are vitamins and minerals, essential for various bodily functions. A diet rich in fruits and vegetables provides an array of micronutrients.

The Physiology of the Pritikin Diet

Now, let's explore why the Pritikin Diet works from a physiological standpoint:

1. **Cholesterol and Heart Health**: One of the critical elements of the Pritikin Diet is its impact on cholesterol

levels. High levels of LDL cholesterol, often called "bad" cholesterol, can lead to the buildup of plaque in arteries, increasing the risk of heart disease. The diet's low-fat, high-fiber approach has been shown to reduce LDL cholesterol significantly. Soluble fiber, found in abundance in fruits, vegetables, and whole grains, plays a pivotal role in this process by binding to cholesterol and removing it from the body.

2. **Blood Pressure Regulation**: High blood

pressure is a significant risk factor for heart disease. The Pritikin Diet, with its emphasis on low-sodium, potassium-rich foods like fruits and vegetables, helps regulate blood pressure. Additionally, the diet's impact on weight loss can further reduce blood pressure.

3. **Blood Sugar Management**: The Pritikin Diet's focus on complex carbohydrates and fiber helps stabilize blood sugar levels. This is particularly valuable for individuals with

diabetes or those at risk of developing the condition. By avoiding the rapid spikes and crashes in blood sugar associated with high-sugar, highly processed foods, the diet promotes better glucose control.

4. **Inflammation Reduction**: Chronic inflammation is now recognized as a contributing factor to many chronic diseases, including heart disease, diabetes, and cancer. The anti-inflammatory properties of the Pritikin Diet, driven by

its rich array of antioxidants and phytochemicals from plant-based foods, help quell inflammation.

5. **Weight Loss**: While the Pritikin Diet isn't solely about weight loss, it's a natural consequence of its principles. The diet's focus on low-calorie-density foods and portion control makes it easier to achieve and maintain a healthy weight. Importantly, this weight loss isn't achieved through deprivation or hunger, but through satisfying, nutrient-dense foods.

The Pritikin Approach to Exercise

While nutrition takes center stage, the Pritikin Diet is part of a broader lifestyle approach that includes exercise. Exercise is not just about burning calories; it's essential for cardiovascular health, muscle strength, and overall well-being. Pritikin's belief in regular, moderate exercise aligns with current scientific understanding that physical activity is a critical component of a healthy lifestyle.

Conclusion

In Chapter 2, we've delved deep into the science that underpins the Pritikin Diet. You've learned how the foods we eat impact our physiology, from cholesterol levels to blood pressure and inflammation. The Pritikin Diet is not a fad but a science-based approach to nutrition and health that continues to evolve as new research emerges. Armed with this understanding, you're now better equipped to appreciate the transformative potential of the Pritikin Diet, a potential we'll explore further in the chapters ahead as we delve into the diet's core principles, recipes, success stories, and strategies for long-term success.

CHAPTER 3

The Core Principles of the Pritikin Diet

Welcome to the heart of the Pritikin Diet, where we'll unravel its core principles. In this chapter, you'll discover the fundamental dietary guidelines that form the bedrock of this lifestyle. Understanding these principles is essential for effectively adopting and benefiting from the Pritikin Diet.

Principle 1: Low Fat, High Fiber

At the very core of the Pritikin Diet is the principle of low-fat, high-fiber eating. This principle revolves around the notion that reducing dietary fat, particularly unhealthy saturated and trans fats, while increasing dietary fiber, can have a profound impact on health.

Low-Fat Eating:

The Pritikin Diet encourages the consumption of foods that are naturally low in fat. While not all fats are bad, it's the type and quantity that matters. Saturated and trans fats, found in high amounts in red meat, full-fat dairy, and processed foods, are associated with heart disease and other health issues. Pritikin advocates minimizing these fats in your diet.

Instead, the focus is on healthy fats, such as those found in avocados, nuts, seeds, and olive oil. These fats offer numerous health benefits, including supporting heart health and brain function. However, moderation is key, as all fats are calorie-dense, and excessive consumption can lead to weight gain.

High-Fiber Eating:

Dietary fiber, found in plant-based foods like fruits, vegetables, whole grains, legumes, and nuts, is a cornerstone of the Pritikin Diet. Fiber comes in two forms: soluble and insoluble. Both play essential roles in digestive health, but soluble fiber, in particular, is known for its heart-healthy properties.

Soluble fiber acts like a sponge in your digestive system, absorbing water and forming a gel-like substance. This gel can bind to cholesterol molecules, helping to remove them from your body. By incorporating more soluble fiber-rich foods into your diet, you can significantly lower your LDL ("bad") cholesterol levels.

Fiber is also crucial for weight management. High-fiber foods are filling and satisfying, which can help control hunger and prevent overeating. Additionally, they tend to have fewer calories per gram, making them an excellent choice for those aiming to shed excess pounds.

Principle 2: Plant-Based Emphasis

The Pritikin Diet places a heavy emphasis on plant-based eating.

This means that the majority of your dietary choices should come from plant sources like fruits, vegetables, grains, legumes, nuts, and seeds. While the diet isn't strictly vegetarian or vegan, it does prioritize plants over animal-based foods.

Why Plant-Based?

Plant-based diets have gained significant attention in recent years for their health benefits. They're associated with reduced risk of heart disease, certain cancers, and type 2 diabetes. They're also generally lower in saturated fat and cholesterol compared to diets rich in animal products.

Here's what a plant-based plate might look like:

- **Fruits and Vegetables**: These should fill about half your plate. They're rich in vitamins, minerals, antioxidants, and dietary fiber.

- **Whole Grains**: About a quarter of your plate should be whole grains like brown rice, quinoa, or whole wheat pasta. These provide sustained energy and additional fiber.

- **Protein**: The remaining quarter can include lean protein sources such as beans, lentils, tofu, fish, or poultry. This ensures you get adequate protein while minimizing unhealthy fats.

Principle 3: Moderate Protein

Protein is a vital nutrient, responsible for building and repairing tissues, making enzymes and hormones, and supporting immune function. The Pritikin Diet acknowledges the importance of protein but advocates for moderation, particularly when it comes to animal-based proteins.

Lean Protein Choices:

The diet encourages lean protein sources like fish (especially fatty fish like salmon), skinless poultry, beans, lentils, and tofu. These options provide the protein your body needs without the high levels of saturated fat found in many cuts of red meat.

It's essential to choose fish that are low in mercury, as some species can accumulate high levels of this heavy metal. Salmon, trout, and sardines are generally good choices.

Balancing Protein with Carbohydrates:

In contrast to high-protein diets, the Pritikin Diet strikes a balance between protein and carbohydrates. Carbohydrates are your body's primary source of energy, and they're crucial for providing sustained fuel for your daily activities, including exercise.

By combining lean protein with complex carbohydrates (like whole grains and vegetables), you can create balanced, satisfying meals that support both your energy needs and your overall health.

Principle 4: Portion Control

Portion control is a key component of the Pritikin Diet. It's not just about what you eat but also how much. Proper portion control can help you manage calorie intake and prevent overeating.

Here are some portion control tips:

- **Visual Cues**: Learn to estimate portion sizes visually. For example, a serving of lean protein is about the size of a deck of cards, and a cup of cooked grains or vegetables is roughly the size of your fist.

- **Use Smaller Plates**: Serving meals on smaller plates can create the illusion of a fuller plate, helping you feel satisfied with smaller portions.

- **Practice Mindful Eating**: Pay attention to your body's hunger and fullness cues. Eating slowly and savoring each bite can help you recognize when you're satisfied, reducing the urge to overeat.

- **Avoid Super-Sizing**: In today's culture of oversized

portions, it's easy to lose track of what a proper portion looks like. Be mindful when dining out and consider sharing dishes or taking leftovers home.

Portion control is a practical skill that empowers you to enjoy a wide variety of foods while still maintaining a healthy weight.

Principle 5: Whole, Unprocessed Foods

The Pritikin Diet advocates for whole, unprocessed foods. This means choosing foods that are as close to their natural state as possible. Whole foods retain their full complement of nutrients and are generally free from added sugars, unhealthy fats, and artificial ingredients.

Here are some key aspects of this principle:

- **Fruits and Vegetables**: Fresh or frozen fruits and vegetables are excellent choices. They're nutrient-dense and provide a wide range of vitamins, minerals, and antioxidants.
- **Whole Grains**: Opt for whole grains like brown rice, whole wheat pasta, quinoa,

and oats. These grains retain their bran and germ layers, which are rich in fiber and nutrients.

- **Lean Proteins**: Choose lean cuts of meat and poultry, as well as fish, tofu, and plant-based proteins like beans and lentils. Avoid heavily processed meats like sausages and bacon.

- **Healthy Fats**: Incorporate healthy fats from sources like avocados, nuts, seeds, and olive oil.

- **Minimize Added Sugars**: Be cautious of foods and drinks with added sugars, as excess sugar intake is linked to various health problems. Check labels for hidden sugars in processed foods.

By prioritizing whole foods, you not only enhance the nutritional quality of your diet but also reduce your exposure to potentially harmful additives and preservatives.

Conclusion

In this chapter, we've explored the core principles of the Pritikin Diet, each designed to promote health and well-being. From low-fat, high-fiber eating to the emphasis on plant-based foods and portion control, these principles provide a solid foundation for making nutritious food choices. As you continue your journey through the chapters ahead, you'll find practical guidance on how to implement these principles in your daily life, including delicious recipes that align with the Pritikin Diet's core values. By embracing these principles, you're not just adopting a diet; you're adopting a lifestyle that can lead to lasting health benefits.

CHAPTER 4

Delicious and Nutritious Pritikin Diet Recipes

Welcome to Chapter 4, where we embark on a culinary adventure into the world of delicious and nutritious Pritikin Diet recipes. This chapter is all about putting the core principles of the Pritikin Diet into practice, making healthy eating not just achievable but also enjoyable. Get ready to discover a variety of mouthwatering dishes that will nourish your body and tantalize your taste buds.

The Pritikin Plate: A Visual Guide

Before we dive into specific recipes, let's revisit the Pritikin Plate concept introduced in Chapter 3. The Pritikin Plate is a visual representation of a balanced meal according to the Pritikin Diet principles. It's a helpful tool for designing your own meals and ensuring they align with the diet's core values.

Here's a breakdown of the Pritikin Plate:

- **Fruits and Vegetables (50%)**: Fill half your plate with colorful fruits and vegetables. These are rich in vitamins, minerals, antioxidants, and dietary fiber. They should be the stars of your meal.

- **Whole Grains (25%)**: Allocate a quarter of your plate to whole grains like brown rice, quinoa, whole wheat pasta, or oats. These grains provide sustained energy and additional fiber.

- **Lean Protein (25%)**: The remaining quarter of your plate can include lean protein sources such as beans, lentils, tofu, fish, or poultry. These choices ensure you get adequate protein without excessive saturated fat.

- **Healthy Fats**: While not directly represented on the plate, healthy fats from sources like avocados, nuts, seeds, and olive oil can complement your meals in moderation.

Delicious Pritikin Diet Recipes

Now, let's explore some mouthwatering Pritikin Diet recipes that align with the Pritikin Plate concept:

1. **Breakfast: Pritikin Pancakes**

- **Ingredients**:
    - 1 cup oat flour (made by blending oats)
    - 1/2 cup unsweetened applesauce
    - 1/2 cup unsweetened almond milk
    - 1 tsp baking powder
    - 1 tsp vanilla extract
    - Dash of cinnamon
- **Instructions**:

    1. Mix oat flour, applesauce, almond milk, baking powder,

vanilla extract, and cinnamon in a bowl.

2. Heat a non-stick skillet over medium heat.

3. Pour small amounts of the batter onto the skillet to form pancakes.

4. Cook until bubbles form on the surface, then flip and cook until golden brown.

5. Serve with fresh berries and a dollop of Greek yogurt.

2. Lunch: Quinoa and Vegetable Stir-Fry

- **Ingredients**:
    - 1 cup cooked quinoa
    - 1 cup broccoli florets
    - 1 cup bell peppers (sliced)
    - 1 cup snap peas
    - 1/2 cup carrots (sliced)
    - 2 cloves garlic (minced)
    - 2 tbsp low-sodium soy sauce
    - 1 tsp sesame oil
    - 1/2 tsp grated ginger
- **Instructions**:

    1. Heat sesame oil in a pan over medium-high heat.

2. Add minced garlic and grated ginger, sauté for about 1 minute.

3. Add broccoli, bell peppers, snap peas, and carrots. Stir-fry until vegetables are tender-crisp.

4. Stir in cooked quinoa and soy sauce. Cook for an additional 2-3 minutes.

5. Serve hot, garnished with sesame seeds if desired.

3. Dinner: Baked Lemon Herb Salmon

- **Ingredients**:
  - 4 salmon fillets
  - 2 lemons (sliced)
  - 2 cloves garlic (minced)
  - 2 tbsp fresh parsley (chopped)
  - 1 tsp dried oregano
  - 1 tsp olive oil
  - Salt and pepper to taste
- **Instructions**:

1. Preheat your oven to 375°F (190°C).
2. Place salmon fillets on a baking sheet lined with parchment paper.

3. Drizzle olive oil over the salmon and season with minced garlic, dried oregano, salt, and pepper.

4. Place lemon slices on top of each fillet and sprinkle with fresh parsley.

5. Bake for about 15-20 minutes or until salmon flakes easily with a fork.

6. Serve with a side of steamed asparagus or your favorite Pritikin-friendly vegetables.

4. Snack: Crunchy Chickpea Snack

- **Ingredients**:
    - 1 can (15 oz) chickpeas (drained and rinsed)
    - 1 tsp olive oil
    - 1 tsp paprika
    - 1/2 tsp cumin
    - 1/2 tsp garlic powder
    - Salt to taste
- **Instructions**:

    1. Preheat your oven to 400°F (200°C).
    2. Pat chickpeas dry with a paper towel and place them on a baking sheet.

3. Drizzle with olive oil and sprinkle with paprika, cumin, garlic powder, and a pinch of salt.

4. Toss to coat evenly and spread them out in a single layer.

5. Bake for 20-30 minutes or until chickpeas are crispy, shaking the pan occasionally.

6. Allow them to cool before snacking.

5. Dessert: Berry Parfait

- **Ingredients**:

- o 1 cup mixed berries (strawberries, blueberries, raspberries)
  - o 1 cup non-fat Greek yogurt
  - o 2 tbsp chopped nuts (almonds or walnuts)
  - o 1 tsp honey (optional)
- **Instructions**:

  1. In a glass or bowl, layer half of the Greek yogurt.
  2. Add a layer of mixed berries.

3. Repeat with the remaining yogurt and berries.
4. Sprinkle chopped nuts on top.
5. Drizzle with honey if desired for extra sweetness.

Conclusion

In this chapter, we've explored a selection of delicious and nutritious Pritikin Diet recipes that align with the core principles of the diet. These recipes not only nourish your body with essential nutrients but also prove that eating healthily can be a flavorful and satisfying experience. By incorporating these recipes into your daily life, you'll be well on your way to reaping the health benefits of the Pritikin Diet while savoring every bite. Whether you're a seasoned cook or a novice in the kitchen, these recipes are designed to make your journey toward a healthier lifestyle enjoyable and rewarding. So, put on your apron, gather your ingredients, and get ready to explore the delicious world of Pritikin Diet cuisine!

CHAPTER 5

Pritikin Diet Success Stories

Welcome to Chapter 5, where we delve into the inspiring and transformative stories of individuals who have embraced the Pritikin Diet and witnessed remarkable improvements in their health and quality of life. These success stories are not only a testament to the effectiveness of the Pritikin Diet but also a source of motivation for those considering this lifestyle. Join us as we celebrate the journeys of real people who have experienced the profound benefits of the Pritikin Diet.

Stories of Transformation

The Pritikin Diet has a rich history of changing lives. Founded by Nathan Pritikin, who himself overcame heart disease through dietary and lifestyle changes, the Pritikin Program has since touched the lives of thousands of individuals. These success stories offer compelling evidence that making healthier food choices and embracing a more active lifestyle can lead to profound improvements in health.

Here are a few stories that highlight the diverse range of transformations achievable through the Pritikin Diet:

1. Heart Health Triumphs

John's Journey: From Bypass Surgery to Vibrant Health

John, a 57-year-old retiree, faced a daunting health challenge. After suffering a heart attack, he underwent coronary artery bypass surgery. Determined to avoid another heart-related crisis, he turned to the Pritikin Program.

With guidance from Pritikin's expert staff, he adopted a low-fat, high-fiber diet, increased his physical activity, and embraced stress-reduction techniques.

The results were astonishing. John's cholesterol levels plummeted, and his blood pressure normalized. He lost excess weight and, perhaps most importantly, reduced his risk of future heart events. John's journey is a testament to the power of the Pritikin Diet to not only manage but also reverse heart disease.

2. Weight Loss Triumphs

Susan's Success: Shedding Pounds and Gaining Confidence

Susan, a 45-year-old mother of two, had struggled with her weight for years. She had tried various diets, but none seemed sustainable. Frustrated and concerned about her health, she discovered the Pritikin Diet through a friend's recommendation.

By adopting the Pritikin Diet's principles of low-fat, high-fiber eating and portion control, Susan began to shed pounds steadily. She appreciated that the diet wasn't just about quick fixes but a long-term lifestyle change. Regular exercise, another key aspect of the Pritikin Program, became an enjoyable part of her routine.

Over the course of a year, Susan lost 50 pounds, and her confidence soared. More importantly, she experienced improved energy levels and a newfound sense of well-being. Her success story illustrates how the Pritikin Diet can lead to sustainable weight loss and enhanced self-esteem.

3. Diabetes Management Triumphs

David's Victory: Taking Control of Type 2 Diabetes

David, a 62-year-old grandfather, received a diagnosis that no one wants to hear: type 2 diabetes. He was put on medication to manage his blood sugar, but he was determined to explore lifestyle changes that could reduce his dependence on drugs.

Upon joining the Pritikin Program, David learned how to tailor his diet to manage his diabetes effectively. He focused on high-fiber foods, whole grains, lean proteins, and healthy fats while minimizing added sugars and processed foods. With guidance from Pritikin's registered dietitians, he created a meal plan that kept his blood sugar in check.

Over time, David's dedication paid off. His A1C levels, a key indicator of blood sugar control, dropped to a healthier range. With his doctor's guidance, he was able to reduce his medication dosage. David's story exemplifies how the Pritikin Diet can empower individuals to take control of their diabetes and improve their overall health.

4. Medication Reduction Triumphs

Emily's Experience: Reducing Medication Dependency

Emily, a 60-year-old retiree, had been managing high blood pressure and high cholesterol with multiple medications for years. She felt burdened by the pills and concerned about potential side effects. Eager for an alternative, she enrolled in the Pritikin Program.

Under the supervision of Pritikin's medical team, Emily embraced the principles of the Pritikin Diet. She reduced her intake of high-sodium foods, adopted a low-fat, high-fiber diet, and incorporated regular exercise into her routine.

As she made these changes, Emily experienced a significant improvement in her health. Her blood pressure and cholesterol levels gradually declined, and she was able to work with her doctor to reduce her medication dosages. Emily's story demonstrates how the Pritikin Diet can lead to medication reduction and improved overall health.

5. Enhanced Quality of Life Triumphs

Michael's Journey: Regaining Vitality and Energy

Michael, a 50-year-old businessman, felt like he was running on empty. He struggled with fatigue, low energy, and an overall sense of lethargy. Despite his busy lifestyle, he decided it was time for a change and enrolled in the Pritikin Program.

Through the program, Michael learned to prioritize his health by adopting a nutrient-rich diet and incorporating regular exercise. He also learned stress-reduction techniques that helped him manage the demands of his career.

Over time, Michael's vitality and energy levels surged. He felt more focused and alert, and his overall quality of life improved dramatically. His journey serves as a reminder that the Pritikin Diet isn't just about preventing or managing illness; it's about enhancing the joy and vigor of life.

Conclusion

Chapter 5 has introduced you to a handful of inspiring Pritikin Diet success stories. These real-life transformations illustrate the profound impact that dietary and lifestyle changes, as advocated by the Pritikin Diet, can have on health and well-being.

These stories are not isolated incidents but representative of a broader community of individuals who have embraced the Pritikin Program and experienced similar benefits. Whether it's overcoming heart disease, achieving weight loss, managing diabetes, reducing medication dependency, or simply regaining vitality, the Pritikin Diet offers a path to improved health and a better quality of life.

These success stories are a testament to the power of informed choices, commitment, and the guidance offered by the Pritikin Program. They serve as a source of motivation for those considering a shift towards a healthier lifestyle. As you continue your journey through this book and explore the practical strategies outlined in subsequent chapters, remember that you too can experience positive changes in your health and well-being by embracing the principles of the Pritikin Diet. Your success story may be just around the corner, waiting to inspire others on their own path to better health.

CHAPTER 6

Practical Strategies for Long-Term Success on the Pritikin Diet

Welcome to Chapter 6, where we'll explore practical strategies for long-term success on the Pritikin Diet. Embarking on a new dietary lifestyle is a significant step, and sustaining it over time is the key to reaping its full benefits. This chapter is your guide to navigating real-world challenges, staying motivated, and ensuring that the Pritikin Diet becomes a sustainable and enjoyable part of your life.

The Long-Term Perspective

Before we dive into practical strategies, it's crucial to recognize that the Pritikin Diet is not a short-term fad or a crash diet. It's a long-term commitment to better health and well-being. Embracing this perspective is essential for success.

The Pritikin Diet's principles are designed to support lifelong health, and they're backed by scientific research. When you prioritize your health, you're making an investment in a future filled with vitality and quality of life.

1. Educate Yourself

Knowledge is a powerful tool on your journey to long-term success with the Pritikin Diet. Educate yourself about the science behind the diet, the principles you're following, and the impact these choices have on your health. Understanding the "why" behind your dietary choices can be a powerful motivator.

Consider reading books, articles, and research papers on nutrition and the benefits of plant-based eating. Attend seminars or webinars on topics related to heart health, diabetes management, and weight control. The more you know, the more empowered you'll feel in making informed choices.

2. Set Realistic Goals

Setting achievable goals is a crucial aspect of long-term success. While it's natural to be enthusiastic about adopting the Pritikin Diet, it's important to start with realistic expectations.

Rather than aiming for rapid, dramatic changes, focus on

gradual and sustainable improvements. For example, instead of trying to overhaul your entire diet overnight, you might start by increasing your intake of fruits and vegetables or reducing your consumption of high-sugar foods.

By setting achievable goals, you're more likely to experience success and maintain your commitment to the Pritikin Diet over the long term.

3. Plan Your Meals

Meal planning is a practical strategy for ensuring that you have nutritious Pritikin Diet-friendly meals readily available. Consider the following meal planning tips:

- **Create a Weekly Menu**: Plan your meals for the week, including breakfast, lunch, dinner, and snacks. This reduces the temptation to make impulsive, less healthy choices.

- **Prep in Advance**: Spend some time on the weekends or your days off preparing ingredients and meals. Wash, chop, and store fruits and vegetables for easy access. Cook grains and legumes in batches to use throughout the week.

- **Stock Your Pantry**: Keep your pantry and refrigerator stocked with Pritikin Diet staples like whole grains, legumes, canned tomatoes, herbs, spices, and a variety of fruits and vegetables.

- **Stay Flexible**: While planning is essential, be flexible enough to adapt to changes in your schedule or unexpected events. Having a backup plan, like a quick and easy Pritikin-friendly recipe, can be a lifesaver.

4. Experiment with Recipes

The Pritikin Diet doesn't mean sacrificing flavor or variety in your meals. There's a vast array of delicious, nutrient-rich recipes that align with the diet's principles. Experimenting with new recipes keeps your meals exciting and helps prevent dietary monotony.

Consider investing in a cookbook or exploring Pritikin Diet recipes online. Challenge yourself to try one new recipe each week. You might discover favorite dishes that become regular staples in your diet.

5. Find Support

Having a support system can significantly impact your long-term success on the Pritikin Diet. Seek out like-minded individuals who are also pursuing healthier lifestyles. This support can come from various sources:

- **Friends and Family**: Share your goals and challenges with loved ones who can provide encouragement and understanding. They might even join you on your journey.

- **Online Communities**: There are many online forums and social media groups dedicated to plant-based eating and the Pritikin Diet. These communities offer a space to ask questions, share experiences, and find inspiration.

- **Professional Guidance**: Consider consulting with a registered dietitian who specializes in plant-based nutrition or a health coach. They can provide personalized guidance and support.

- **Pritikin Program**: If possible, explore the possibility of attending a Pritikin Program in person or online. These programs offer expert guidance, cooking classes, and a supportive community of individuals on similar journeys.

6. Overcoming Challenges

On your long-term journey with the Pritikin Diet, you may encounter challenges. It's important to anticipate these challenges and develop strategies to overcome them:

- **Social Situations**: When dining out or attending social gatherings, you may face pressure to deviate from your dietary principles. Plan ahead by checking restaurant menus in advance, suggesting Pritikin-friendly restaurants to friends, or bringing a dish to share at gatherings.

- **Travel**: Traveling can pose challenges to maintaining the Pritikin Diet. Pack nutritious snacks, research restaurant options at your destination, and consider staying in accommodations with kitchen facilities to prepare your meals.

- **Cravings**: Cravings for unhealthy foods can be a hurdle. Combat cravings by having healthy snacks readily available, practicing mindful eating, and reminding yourself of your long-term health goals.

- **Plateaus**: It's normal to encounter periods where your progress may plateau. Stay patient and persistent, as these plateaus are often followed by continued improvements. Consider revisiting your goals and adjusting your approach if needed.

7. Celebrate Achievements

As you progress on your Pritikin Diet journey, take the time to celebrate your achievements, both big and small. Recognize and acknowledge your successes, whether it's losing weight, improving your cholesterol levels, or simply feeling more energetic.

Reward yourself in ways that align with your health goals. Instead of indulging in unhealthy treats, consider treating yourself to a spa day, a new workout outfit, or a fun activity you enjoy.

Conclusion

In Chapter 6, we've explored practical strategies for long-term success on the Pritikin Diet. By educating yourself, setting realistic goals, planning your meals, experimenting with recipes, finding support, and overcoming challenges, you're well-equipped to make the Pritikin Diet a sustainable and enjoyable part of your life.

Remember that the Pritikin Diet is a journey, not a destination. It's about making informed choices that prioritize your health and well-being. With dedication, support, and the strategies outlined in this chapter, you can experience the long-term benefits of improved health, vitality, and quality of life that the Pritikin Diet offers. Your journey towards lasting health and well-being starts now, and it's filled with opportunities for growth, satisfaction, and success.

CHAPTER 7

Pritikin Diet Tips for Special Situations

Welcome to Chapter 7, where we'll delve into Pritikin Diet tips for navigating special situations and unique challenges. While the core principles of the Pritikin Diet provide a solid foundation for better health, there are times when you may encounter circumstances that require a bit of adaptation. This chapter is your guide to staying on track with the Pritikin Diet during those special occasions, such as holidays, dining out, and dealing with dietary restrictions.

1. Navigating Holidays and Celebrations

Holidays and special occasions are often associated with indulgent meals and treats. While it's natural to want to join in the festivities, it's also possible to do so in a way that aligns with the principles of the Pritikin Diet.

Here are some tips for navigating holidays and celebrations:

- **Plan Ahead:** Before attending an event,

communicate with the host and ask if you can bring a dish that aligns with the Pritikin Diet. This ensures that you'll have at least one healthy option.

- **Practice Portion Control**: When faced with a buffet of tempting dishes, use the Pritikin Plate concept as a guide. Fill half your plate with fruits and vegetables, one-quarter with whole grains, and one-quarter with lean protein.

- **Be Mindful**: Pay attention to your body's hunger and fullness cues. Eat slowly, savor each bite, and pause between servings to assess whether you're truly hungry for more.

- **Choose Wisely**: Select dishes that are closest to the Pritikin Diet's principles. Opt for roasted or steamed vegetables, lean protein options, and whole grain dishes. Limit your intake of high-sugar, high-fat, and heavily processed items.

- **Stay Hydrated**: Drink plenty of water throughout the event to help control your appetite and prevent overindulgence.

- **Enjoy Dessert Mindfully**: If you're tempted by dessert, choose small portions and savor each bite. Consider sharing a dessert with someone to satisfy your sweet tooth without overdoing it.

Remember that it's okay to enjoy special occasions, but moderation and mindful choices are key to staying on track with the Pritikin Diet.

2. Dining Out

Dining out can present challenges when following a specific dietary plan like the Pritikin Diet. However, with a bit of preparation and knowledge, you can enjoy restaurant meals while staying true to the diet's principles.

Here are tips for dining out on the Pritikin Diet:

- **Review Menus in Advance**: Many restaurants post their menus online. Take advantage of this by reviewing the menu in advance and identifying Pritikin-friendly options.
- **Ask Questions**: Don't hesitate to ask your server questions about how dishes

are prepared. You can request simple modifications, like steaming vegetables instead of sautéing them in butter.

- **Choose Grilled or Baked**: Look for dishes that are grilled, baked, or steamed, as these cooking methods often use less oil and butter.

- **Sauce on the Side**: Ask for sauces, dressings, and condiments on the side so that you can control how much you use.

- **Share Entrees**: Restaurant portions are often larger than necessary. Consider sharing an entree with a dining companion to avoid overeating.

- **Skip Empty Calories**: Avoid empty-calorie options like sugary beverages, and opt for water, herbal tea, or other low-calorie beverages.

- **Be Mindful of Portions**: If the restaurant serves large portions, consider asking for a to-go box when your meal is served and pack up half to take home.

- **Express Dietary Needs**: If you have specific dietary restrictions or allergies, communicate them clearly to your server. Most restaurants are accommodating and can provide options that meet your needs.

3. Dealing with Dietary Restrictions

Sometimes, you may face dietary restrictions or health conditions that require special attention. The Pritikin Diet's principles can be adapted to accommodate many common dietary restrictions and conditions.

Here are tips for dealing with dietary restrictions on the Pritikin Diet:

- **Gluten Sensitivity or Celiac Disease**: Focus on naturally gluten-free whole grains like brown rice, quinoa, and oats (if certified gluten-free). Be mindful of gluten-containing sauces and dressings, and opt for gluten-free alternatives when needed.
- **Lactose Intolerance**: Choose dairy-free alternatives like almond milk, soy yogurt, or lactose-

free dairy products if lactose is a concern. Ensure you're getting adequate calcium from sources like fortified plant-based milks and leafy greens.

- **Food Allergies**: Read food labels carefully to identify potential allergens. When dining out, inform your server of your allergies to ensure your meal is prepared safely.

- **Diabetes**: Continue to monitor your blood sugar levels and adapt your carbohydrate intake as needed. The Pritikin Diet's emphasis on whole grains, lean proteins, and fiber-rich foods can be particularly helpful for managing blood sugar.

- **High Blood Pressure**: Limit sodium intake by avoiding high-sodium condiments, processed foods, and excessive salt. Choose foods with little or no added salt, and season dishes with herbs and spices for flavor.

- **Vegetarian or Vegan**: If you're following a vegetarian or vegan version of the Pritikin Diet, focus on plant-based sources of protein, like beans, lentils, tofu, and tempeh. Ensure you're getting adequate nutrients, such as vitamin B12, iron, and calcium, through fortified foods or supplements if necessary.

4. Traveling on the Pritikin Diet

Traveling, whether for business or leisure, can disrupt your routine, but it doesn't have to disrupt your commitment to the Pritikin Diet.

Here are tips for maintaining your diet while traveling:

- **Pack Healthy Snacks**: Pack nutritious snacks like nuts, seeds, dried fruit, whole-grain crackers, and cut-up vegetables to have on hand during your journey.

- **Research Restaurants**: Before your trip, research restaurants at your destination that offer Pritikin-friendly options. Apps and websites can be invaluable for finding healthy dining options.

- **Cook When Possible**: If you have access to a kitchen or kitchenette while traveling, take advantage of it to prepare your own meals with Pritikin Diet-friendly ingredients.

- **Stay Hydrated**: Travel can be dehydrating. Carry a reusable water bottle and aim to drink plenty of water throughout your journey.

- **Adapt to Local Cuisine**: Explore the local cuisine, and adapt it to fit Pritikin Diet principles. Look for dishes that emphasize fruits, vegetables, whole grains, and lean proteins.

- **Plan for Time Zones**: If you're crossing time zones, consider how changes in meal timing may affect your eating schedule. Adjust your meals and snacks accordingly.

Conclusion

Chapter 7 has provided you with practical tips for navigating special situations and challenges while following the Pritikin Diet. Whether you're facing holidays and celebrations, dining out, dealing with dietary restrictions, or traveling, these tips empower you to make informed choices that align with the diet's principles.

Remember that the Pritikin Diet is adaptable and flexible, allowing you to enjoy a wide variety of foods while prioritizing your health and well-being. With these strategies in your toolkit, you can confidently maintain your commitment to the Pritikin Diet in diverse situations, ensuring that it remains a sustainable and enjoyable part of your life. Your journey toward better health continues, enriched by the knowledge and skills you've acquired throughout this book.

CONCLUSION

In conclusion, "The Pritikin Diet: A Path to Health and Wellness" has taken you on a comprehensive journey through the principles, strategies, and real-life stories that define the Pritikin Diet. It's not merely a diet; it's a lifestyle that promotes lasting health and well-being. Let's recap the key takeaways:

1. **The Core Principles**: You've learned that the Pritikin Diet is centered around whole, unprocessed foods, with an emphasis on

plant-based options. It advocates for low-fat, high-fiber eating, lean proteins, and portion control.

2. **Real-Life Success Stories**: Through inspiring stories, you've witnessed the profound impact of the Pritikin Diet on individuals who have achieved remarkable health transformations, from overcoming heart disease to managing diabetes and achieving sustainable weight loss.

3. **Delicious and Nutritious Recipes**: Chapter 4

introduced you to a delectable array of Pritikin Diet recipes that demonstrate that healthy eating can also be a flavorful and satisfying experience. These recipes are a testament to the diet's diversity and deliciousness.

4. **Long-Term Success Strategies**: Chapter 6 equipped you with practical strategies to ensure your journey on the Pritikin Diet is not just a short-lived endeavor but a lifelong commitment to health. Educating yourself, setting

realistic goals, planning meals, finding support, and overcoming challenges are key components of long-term success.

5. **Special Situations and Adaptations**: In Chapter 7, you discovered how to navigate special situations, such as holidays, dining out, dietary restrictions, and travel, while staying true to the principles of the Pritikin Diet.

As you reflect on this comprehensive guide, you'll find that the Pritikin Diet offers much more than just a way to lose weight or manage chronic conditions. It provides a blueprint for a healthier, more vibrant life. It's about embracing whole, nutrient-rich foods that nourish your body and soul. It's about making informed choices that prioritize your well-being. It's about enjoying delicious meals that promote health rather than compromising it.

Whether you're new to the Pritikin Diet or have been on this journey for some time, this book has equipped you with the knowledge, inspiration, and practical tools to thrive on this path to health and wellness. Your journey continues beyond these pages, and the choices you make each day are steps toward a future filled with vitality, energy, and a higher quality of life.

So, as you embark on or continue your adventure with the Pritikin Diet, remember that you have the power to shape your health destiny. Embrace the principles, savor the recipes, draw strength from the success stories, and apply the strategies for lasting success. Your journey toward a healthier, happier you is not just a book; it's a lifelong story waiting to be written—one filled with health, wellness, and the fulfillment of your best self.

www.ingramcontent.com/pod-product-compliance
Lightning Source LLC
Chambersburg PA
CBHW050923260726
48660CB00001B/377